Women's Strength Unveiled

A Journey Through Pregnancy, Birth & Beyond

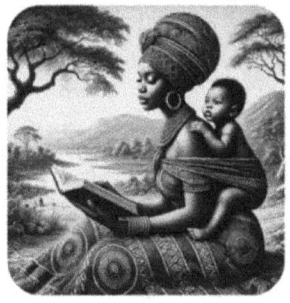

Mahamadou S. Toure

Author & Advocate of Women's Strength

BabouConnect Publishing

Copyright © [2025] Mahamadou S. Toure
All rights reserved.

No part of this book may be reproduced, stored in a retrieval system, or transmitted in any form or by any means—electronic, mechanical, photocopying, recording, or otherwise—without the prior written permission of the publisher, except in the case of brief quotations embodied in critical reviews and certain other noncommercial uses as permitted by copyright law.

Published by: **BabouConnect Publishing**

ISBN: 979-8-9939072-4-6

["Printed in [USA]"]

For permissions, inquiries, or bulk orders, contact:
[**sabilfalah@gmail.com**]

This is a work of nonfiction. The events and figures depicted are based on historical facts, author research, and firsthand accounts. Any errors or omissions are unintentional.

First Edition: [2025]

Men may witness childbirth, but women live it.
This book unveils the strength they carry.

Contents

Introduction: A Journey Into the Unknown.......xiii

Chapter I: The Journey Begins 1
Pregnancy and Its Challenges 1

Chapter II: Labor and Delivery 9
The Crucible of Strength 9
Witnessing the Miracle: 12
A New Perspective on Strength....................12

Chapter III: Childcare 25
The Silent Strength of Women 25
Beyond Resilience 28
Contrast Between a Father's and Mother's Experience of Childbirth 32
The Weight of Motherhood 34

Tribute to Women: The Strength That Deserves Recognition 39

Conclusion: The Unseen Strength of Women..45
Acknowledgments 48

Author's Note..51

To the women who carry **the weight of life,** whose strength remains **unseen but never unfelt**, this book is for you.

Preface

✳ ✳ ✳

Mahamadou S. Toure is a writer, father, and passionate advocate for recognizing the **resilience and sacrifices of women**. With a background in **Public Affairs from Ohio State University**, he brings a unique perspective that blends **personal experience, cultural insight, and social awareness**.

Growing up in West Africa, he witnessed a culture where **pregnancy, labor, and childcare were seen as women's responsibilities**, often with little male involvement. However, his firsthand experience of witnessing childbirth in the United States **transformed his**

perspective and deepened his admiration for women's strength.

Through his writing, Toure explores the **raw realities of pregnancy, labor, and motherhood**, offering a deeply personal yet universal perspective. His work challenges cultural norms, encourages **men to engage more actively in the childbirth experience**, and pays tribute to the **unwavering determination of women**.

As an Author & Advocate of Women's Strength, he believes that **storytelling can bridge cultural perspectives** and highlight the **often-overlooked sacrifices of women**.

Introduction:

A Journey Into the Unknown

Childbirth is often seen as a woman's experience, a journey of endurance, strength, and transformation. But for me, stepping into that world was not just about witnessing birth—it was about discovering something I had never truly understood before.

Where I come from, in West Africa, childbirth happens behind closed doors. Men are not allowed into the labor and delivery ward, and even the women who accompany an expectant mother do not witness the moment of birth. As a result, childbirth is both known and unknown—an event we acknowledge but never truly see.

That was my understanding of birth until I found myself in a delivery room in the United States. Suddenly, I was no longer on the outside. I was inside, standing next to my wife as she endured the unimaginable pain of labor. I watched, helpless yet deeply moved, as she fought through each contraction, driven by love and an instinctive strength I had never witnessed before.

And then came the moment that changed me forever. The nurse handed me a pair of scissors and asked me to cut the umbilical cord. In that instant, I felt the weight of fatherhood settle upon me—not just as a title but as an experience. I realized then that childbirth is not just about bringing life into the world; it is about transformation. It changes a woman. It changes a man. It changes everything.

This book is not just about my experience—it is a tribute to the incredible strength of women. It is a reflection on what I witnessed, what I learned, and how it reshaped my understanding of resilience, love, and sacrifice. Through these pages, I hope to share a story that is both personal and universal—one that highlights the true essence of motherhood, the unseen struggles of childbirth, and the powerful role women play as the backbone of life itself.

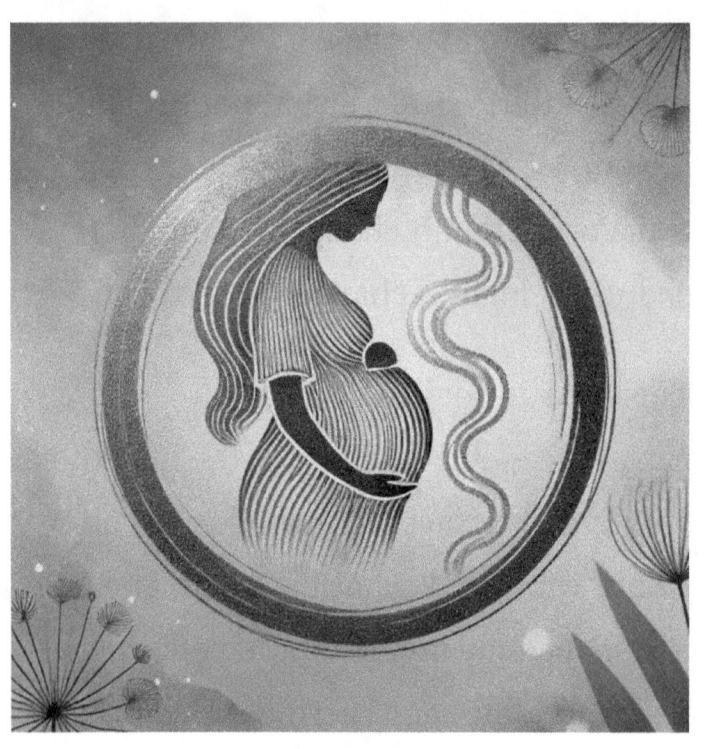

The journey begins!

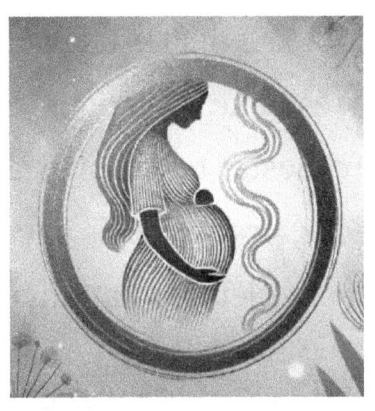

Chapter I:

The Journey Begins

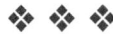

Pregnancy and Its Challenges

Pregnancy is one of the most transformative periods in a woman's life, marked by profound physical and emotional changes. It is a journey of growth—not just for the baby developing in the womb but also for the mother who navigates challenges with remarkable resilience. From the excitement of the first trimester to the physical toll of the final weeks, pregnancy is a testament to the strength and determination of women.

Yet, the experience of pregnancy varies not just from woman to woman, but also across cultures. In my region of West Africa, pregnancy is viewed as a deeply personal and private matter. Men traditionally maintain a respectful distance, showing concern only when absolutely necessary. A husband might ask his wife, "Are you okay?" but rarely goes beyond that. The intricacies of her experience, from morning sickness to fatigue and cravings, often remain unspoken between them. This dynamic is shaped by cultural norms, where pregnancy is considered primarily a woman's domain.

When I moved to the United States, I encountered a very different approach. Here, men are encouraged—and even expected—to be involved throughout the pregnancy journey. They attend doctor's appointments, help track the baby's growth, and participate in decisions about the mother's care. At first, this shift was surprising to me. In my culture, such involvement would have been seen as unnecessary or even intrusive. But as I witnessed it firsthand, I began to understand its importance—not just for the woman but for the family as a whole.

When my wife became pregnant with our first child, I found myself navigating between the cultural norms I grew up with and the expectations of my new environment. At times, I felt unsure of my role. Should I ask more questions? Should I be more involved? My natural instinct was to give her space, as I had seen men do back home. But the more I observed her journey, the more I realized how much support she truly needed. From dealing with nausea and fatigue to managing her emotions, pregnancy was not something she could face alone.

One moment that stands out vividly is when my wife first felt the baby kick. She called me over, placed my hand on her belly, and said, "Feel this." That simple act broke down years of cultural conditioning. It wasn't just her journey—it was ours. I began to ask more questions, to learn more about what she was going through. I realized that being present and involved didn't diminish my respect for her strength; it amplified it.

In my region, men often remain unaware of the details of pregnancy. But through my experience, I've come to see how understanding and participation can strengthen the bond between partners. Pregnancy is not just a physical journey but an emotional and spiritual one, and it deserves the attention and care of both parents.

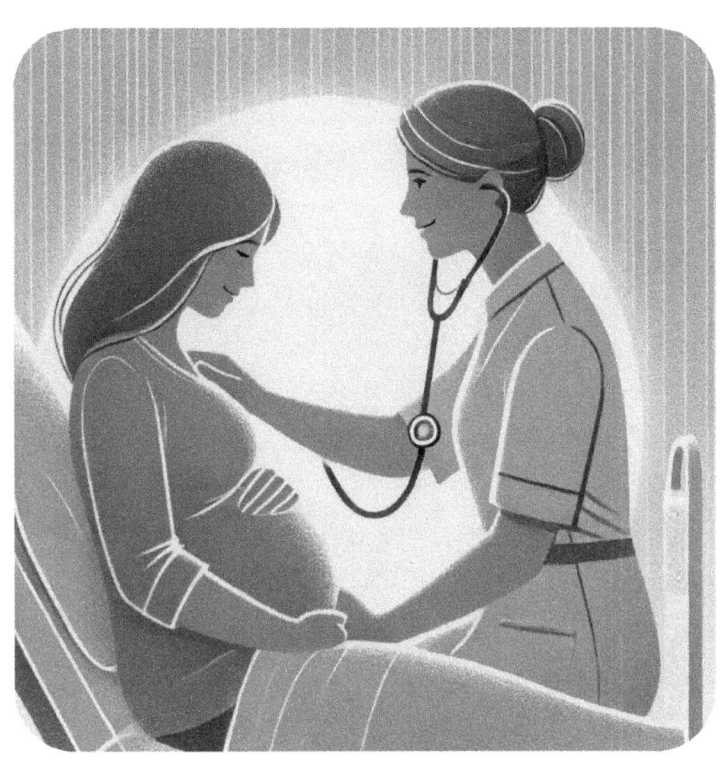

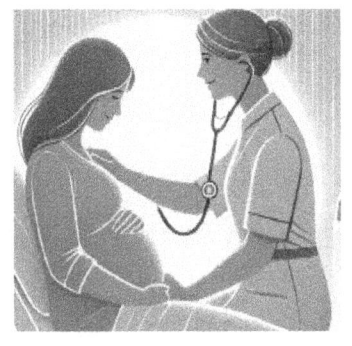

Chapter II:

Labor and Delivery

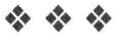

The Crucible of Strength

Labor and delivery stand as one of the most intense and transformative experiences in a woman's life. It is a moment where physical strength, emotional resilience, and an indescribable love converge. The process, though universally shared by women around the world, is deeply personal and shaped by cultural practices and beliefs.

In general terms, labor is divided into stages, each presenting its own challenges and demands. From the early contractions of the first stage to the pushing of the second and the final delivery of the placenta, every moment tests the limits of human endurance. For the woman in labor, it is a journey of pain and perseverance, driven by the hope and love for the life being brought into the world.

Yet, as I have learned, the cultural lens through which labor and delivery are viewed can significantly shape the experience. In my home region of West

Africa, labor is a private matter, often shrouded in mystery for men. Men are strictly forbidden from entering the labor and delivery building, let alone the delivery room. Even women who accompany the expectant mother are not allowed to witness the process firsthand. Only nurses and midwives are permitted inside. As a result, labor becomes an experience shared almost exclusively by the mother and the medical staff, leaving the rest of the family in anxious anticipation outside.

When I moved to the United States, I encountered an entirely different approach. Here, men are not only allowed but encouraged to be present during labor and delivery. They are expected to provide emotional support, advocate for their partners, and witness the birth of their child. At first, this idea felt foreign to me. I couldn't imagine stepping into a space that, in my culture, was considered exclusively for women. But my first experience in the delivery room changed everything.

Witnessing the Miracle: A New Perspective on Streng

1. Mother's Perspective

When my wife went into labor with our first child, **my mother-in-law, who had just arrived from Africa to welcome her first grandchild, accompanied us to the hospital.** Having grown up in a culture where men and even accompanying women were never allowed in the delivery room, **she had little-to-no knowledge of what truly happens behind those closed doors.**

True to her upbringing, she was anxious and unsettled, unable to sit still. She moved from room to room, panicking about what was to come—she had been through it herself but had never witnessed it.

As for me, I initially felt **shy and hesitant, unsure if my presence would be helpful or intrusive.** I wanted to give my wife privacy and space. But as the hours wore on and **my mother-in-law had to step out, overwhelmed by the intensity of the moment,** I found myself in the delivery room alongside my wife, feeling powerless.

I watched as she endured immense pain with **patience and strength, driven by an indescribable love for the life she was bringing into the world.**

Nurses came and went, offering support where they could, but it was my wife who bore the weight of the experience.

After a long labor, my wife battled wave after wave of contractions, displaying a level of strength and patience I had never seen before. Yet the delivery became prolonged, and complications arose, requiring the medical team to use a vacuum to assist the birth. I was overcome with fear and worry when our baby was born with a pyramid-shaped head. I anxiously questioned the nurse about when the baby's head would return to normal, and her reassurance allowed me to breathe again. In that moment, I turned to my wife, who, despite all she had been through, radiated love and care for our child. She seemed to forget the pain almost immediately—a testament to the incredible strength and resilience of women.

2. Nurses' Perspective: Silent Guardians of Birth

In the intensity of labor and delivery, nurses are the unsung heroes. Their patience, honesty, and unwavering dedication make an immeasurable difference in the lives of expectant parents. They are not just medical professionals; they are guides, reassurers, and sometimes the only source of calm in the storm of childbirth.

I witnessed this firsthand when my wife's contractions became relentless, coming back-to-back with little to no pause. Panic crept in, and I could see the fear in her eyes as the pain overwhelmed her. But in that moment, a nurse calmly leaned in, explaining what was happening and why. She spoke in a reassuring tone, letting my wife know that her body was doing exactly what it needed to do, that the baby was on the way. That simple explanation, delivered with patience and kindness, helped ease the panic in the room.

And then came a moment of unexpected joy. As the baby started crowning and her tiny head became visible, a nurse suddenly exclaimed, **"It's a girl!"** Her voice was filled with excitement, and she called for other nurses to come witness the moment. It was as if, for a second, they forgot the intensity of the medical procedure at hand and simply celebrated life. The nurse turned to me with a warm smile and asked, **"Did you know she was a girl?"**

I smiled back, exhaling a deep breath I hadn't realized I was holding. **In that moment, I wasn't just a man standing in a delivery room—I was a father witnessing the first glimpse of my daughter.**

3. Father's Perspective

As a man, witnessing the process of labor and delivery is a humbling experience. It forces you to redefine what strength truly means. While men may possess physical strength—the kind used to fight wars or assert dominance—what I saw in my wife during childbirth was a strength far greater. It was a strength rooted in patience, resilience, and love, the kind that builds life rather than destroys it.

In that moment, I realized something profound: the strength we, as men, often pride ourselves on pales in comparison to the fortitude of women. Their ability to endure pain, push through exhaustion, and still find the capacity to love and nurture is unmatched. It made me reflect on how easily men can misuse their strength, while women channel theirs into creating and sustaining life.

Unexpected

In the midst of all the intensity, something happened that I will never forget. The baby had just been delivered, the nurse was cleaning and tending to the newborn, and then—without any warning—she turned to me and handed me a pair of scissors.

"Go ahead, cut the cord," she said casually, as if it were the most normal thing in the world.

I froze. My mind raced between panic and excitement. What? Me? Right now? My hands hesitated as I took the scissors, staring at the umbilical cord that had been my baby's lifeline for the past nine months. This was the final step before my child would be completely independent from the womb, and I was the one chosen to make that cut.

Culture Shock

It wasn't until a few days after we returned home that I fully realized how unique my experience had been. My mother-in-law and I kept exchanging looks, both of us carrying a mix of shyness and humor. I felt a little ashamed, knowing I had stepped into a space that was traditionally off-limits to men in my culture, while she seemed equally humbled by what she had witnessed.

As the days passed, I couldn't stop thinking about it. I began calling my cousins and brothers who lived abroad, **campaigning with urgency:**

"Don't miss the birth of your first child. Go to the delivery room. Be there for the moment!"

I wanted them to experience what I had a moment that redefined my understanding of strength and love.

Conclusion: Witnessing the process of childbirth not only changes how you view strength but also leaves a lasting impact on how you approach life. For men, being present during such an intense and transformative moment deepens your respect for women in ways you never imagined. It redefines your role as a partner, instills a profound sense of gratitude, and teaches you that the strength of women is not something to be compared but revered.

Labor and delivery are not just the crucible of life but a testament to the unwavering determination and love that only a mother can possess.

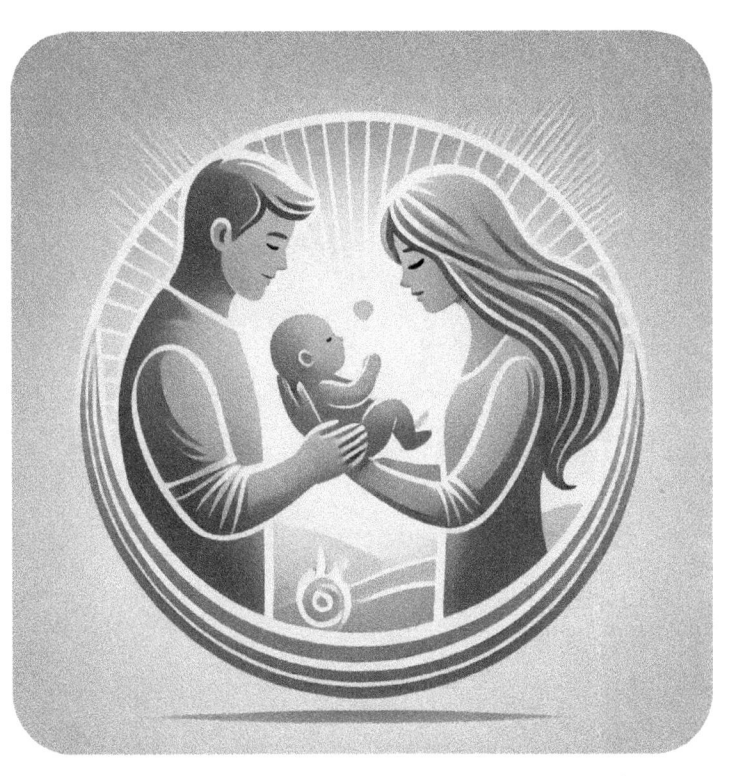

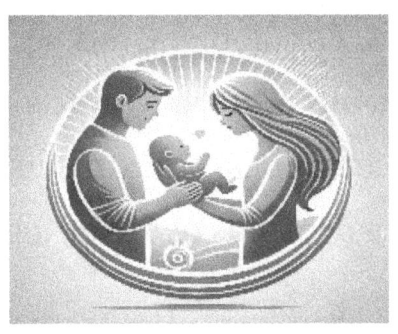

Chapter III:

Childcare

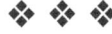

The Silent Strength of Women

If pregnancy and labor are tests of endurance and resilience, childcare is the lifelong marathon that follows. The journey of raising a child begins the moment the baby is born and requires an unyielding combination of patience, love, and selflessness. For mothers, this period often comes with physical recovery from childbirth, emotional adjustments, and the unrelenting demands of caring for a newborn.

In general terms, childcare in the early months revolves around feeding, soothing, and protecting the baby. Sleep becomes a luxury as mothers wake up multiple times during the night to feed or comfort their crying infant. Doctors' appointments, vaccination schedules, and endless diaper changes add to the responsibilities. For women who work outside the home, the challenge is even greater, as they often return to their jobs just a few months after giving birth, balancing professional responsibilities with their roles as caregivers.

In my home region of West Africa, childcare is often seen as the mother's primary responsibility. Extended family members may offer support, but the bulk of the work falls on the mother. Men, though respected as providers, are traditionally less involved in the day-to-day care of their children. This cultural norm can sometimes lead to the perception that childcare is simply "what women do," with little acknowledgment of the sacrifices and strength it demands.

Beyond Resilience

As I reflect on my journey as a father, one of the most profound lessons I've learned is the true depth of resilience and strength that women possess. It's not just their ability to endure the pain of childbirth but their unwavering determination to give and nurture life, even when faced with challenges that would seem insurmountable to others.

After the birth of our third child, who was born prematurely, I witnessed my wife's unwavering determination. Despite the challenges of caring for a fragile newborn, she returned to work full-time, managed our household, and ensured our older children were thriving in school. **Her ability to juggle these responsibilities left me in awe.**

Before the second birthday of our daughters, I began to notice something about my wife. In her quiet moments, when she was talking to her sister or cousin back home, I would often overhear her casually bringing up the idea of having another child. There was a hope in her voice—a yearning, almost—as though she already knew what she wanted: **a boy.**

But for me, those conversations stirred a different set of emotions. Each time I thought about the resilience and strength she had shown during childbirth, I couldn't help but feel hesitant. **I had seen what she endured to bring our daughters into the world—the pain, the sacrifices, the strength it took to push through.** The memory of those moments lingered with me, and I found myself shying away from suggesting another pregnancy. The thought of her going through that experience again, of bearing that kind of pain once more, made me cautious, almost protective.

Still, her determination was undeniable. **She carried this quiet strength, this unwavering belief in her ability to face whatever challenges motherhood brought her way.** And while I hesitated, she stood firm in her hope, undeterred by the sacrifices she knew would come. That kind of strength, that kind of resilience, goes beyond anything I had ever witnessed before.

It is through moments like these that I've come to understand that **resilience is not just about enduring pain or overcoming challenges.** It is about the quiet strength to hope, to love, and to give endlessly, even when the path ahead is uncertain. **For my wife, resilience wasn't a choice—it was simply a part of who she is**, a testament to the incredible strength of women.

Contrast Between a Father's and Mother's Experience of Childbirth

A few months after the birth, I found myself reflecting on everything that had happened in that delivery room. I decided to ask my wife a question, half-serious, half-sarcastic.

"Hey, in that room, who felt the pain more?" I asked with a smirk.

She didn't even hesitate. **"I don't,"** she said flatly.

I laughed, but in that moment, I realized something even deeper. She had gone through so much—hours of labor, unimaginable pain, and exhaustion—and yet, months later, **it was as if the pain had faded into the background.** What remained was her love and the overwhelming joy of motherhood.

Still curious, I pushed further. **"Okay, but what do you actually remember as pain?"** I asked.

She shrugged. **"The wave contractions. That's all."**

I couldn't believe it. After everything she had endured, she summed it up in just two words. I decided to be more playful.

"What men feel in that room is psychological pain, while you feel physical pain," I teased.

She turned to me with a knowing look and simply said, **"No, you can't compare."**

That simple exchange showed me something profound: while I had witnessed every moment of the struggle, **she had lived it.** And yet, her strength wasn't just in enduring pain—**it was in how quickly she moved forward, embracing the journey of motherhood without looking back.**

The Weight of Motherhood

The birth of our son brought its own set of challenges. Born during a time of minimal hospital staffing, his arrival was an event I will never forget. But it was the months that followed that truly deepened my respect for my wife.

She faced each day with resilience, managing the demands of a newborn while continuing to support our family. Her strength became the anchor that held us all together.

Through these experiences, I've come to realize that childcare is more than a responsibility—**it is a reflection of a woman's unmatched dedication and love.** Women are the backbone of the family, not because they are expected to be, but because **they choose to give so much of themselves for the well-being of their children.**

In my culture, where men are often less involved in the nuances of childcare, **it is easy to overlook the depth of a**

mother's sacrifices. But my journey as a husband and father has opened my eyes to the true essence of motherhood. **Women are the silent heroes of every family,** carrying the weight of their children's needs while often neglecting their own.

As I reflect on the strength of the women in my life, I am reminded of a simple yet profound truth: **women are the vehicle of life.** Their love, resilience, and determination form the foundation upon which families are built and thrive. **Childcare is not just a phase in a child's life—it is a testament to the enduring strength and selflessness of women.**

Strength: endurance, love, and sacrifice.

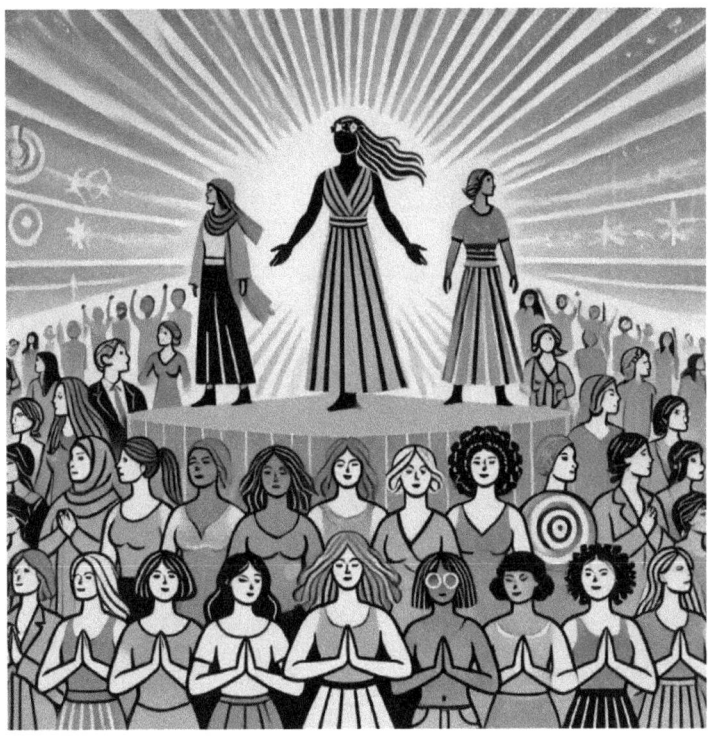

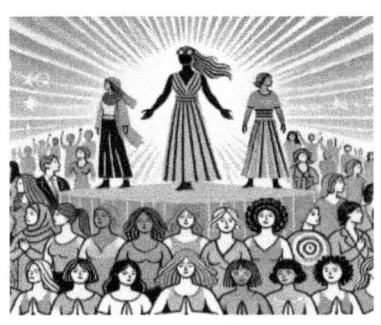

Tribute to Women:

✺ ✺ ✺

The Strength That Deserves Recognition

Throughout history, societies have placed expectations on women—expectations to endure, to nurture, to be the foundation of families and communities. Yet, too often, their sacrifices go unnoticed, and their struggles are met with indifference. It is time to change that.

A woman's resilience is not just in carrying life but in the unseen battles she fights after birth. The world may celebrate the moment of delivery, but what follows is often overlooked—the sleepless nights, the relentless cries of a newborn, the emotional toll of balancing recovery with the weight of new responsibilities. **Women endure all of this while still giving, still nurturing, still holding the family together.**

For this alone, they deserve more than acknowledgment; they deserve **forgiveness** and **patience**. A man may claim physical strength, but what is strength if not the ability to endure? And what is endurance if not the silent sacrifices made without complaint?

In many cultures, including in ancient societies and across Africa, traditions have shaped how men view women. But those traditions must evolve, not to diminish a man's role, but to elevate his understanding. **To the men who hold onto outdated beliefs—ask yourselves: if strength is what defines a person, then who is stronger than the woman who gives life, nourishes it, and carries it forward despite every hardship?**

In my experience, the toughest women during childcare are often those with the most **determination—and determined women have boundless generosity**. They do not endure for themselves; they endure for others. **Their resilience is not just a trait; it is a gift that sustains families, communities, and generations.**

Men must not only **recognize** this strength but also **honor it** with patience, understanding, and unwavering respect. Women do not ask for much—but they deserve everything.

Conclusion:

The Unseen Strength of Women

If there is one truth that stands out above all, it is this: **women are the essence of life, the silent pillars upon which families and societies are built.**

From the moment of pregnancy, through the trials of labor, and into the endless journey of childcare, women display a strength that is often unseen, unspoken, and underappreciated. Their endurance is not just in the pain they bear but in the love they give, the sacrifices they make, and the resilience they embody every single day.

This book has been a journey—a reflection on what I have witnessed, what I have learned, and what I have come to deeply understand. Childbirth is not just a medical event; it is a moment that transforms a woman, challenges a man, and reshapes the very foundation of a family. It is a test of endurance, not just for the mother but for everyone who bears witness to her strength.

For generations, women have carried these burdens with little recognition. Yet, **to truly understand their strength is to honor it—to acknowledge their sacrifices, their struggles, and their unwavering love.**

Through these pages, I have sought to unveil what often goes unseen—to give voice to the resilience of women and to shed light on the depth of their role in shaping life itself.

May this book serve as a reminder, a tribute, and a source of understanding for those who read it.

Acknowledgments

I would like to express my deepest gratitude to those who have supported me throughout this journey. To my family—your unwavering belief in my vision has been my greatest source of strength. To my wife, whose resilience and love inspired much of this book, and to my children, who remind me daily of the beauty and responsibility of parenthood—thank you.

To the women who shared their stories, knowingly or unknowingly, shaping my understanding of the strength, sacrifice, and determination that define motherhood—I dedicate this work to you.

To my readers, thank you for taking the time to explore this journey with me. If this book has resonated with you, it is because the truth of women's resilience is universal.

Author's Note

A Personal Reflection

When I first witnessed childbirth, it changed everything I thought I knew. I saw pain, patience, and ultimately, a love so powerful it could only be described as **the purest strength**. This book is my way of sharing that experience, of giving words to the awe I felt in that moment.

In many cultures, the challenges of pregnancy, labor, and childcare are expected of women but rarely spoken about in depth. Their sacrifices are **felt but often overlooked**. I hope this book encourages

greater awareness, respect, and appreciation for the resilience of women.

For men, I hope it serves as an invitation—to witness, to understand, and to support. **We don't have to experience childbirth to respect the depth of its strength.** We just have to be willing to see, listen, and acknowledge.

Final Thought

If this book has moved you, I encourage you to share its message. **Talk about it, discuss it, challenge cultural perceptions.** Conversations about the strength of women should not be confined to women alone.

Change begins with awareness and action. Whether you are a parent, a spouse, a son, or simply someone willing to listen, you have a role to play in honoring and supporting the women in your life.

A mother's strength does not fade after labor—it carries through every sleepless night, every sacrificed moment, and every act of care. Let us recognize, appreciate, and advocate for that strength—not just in words, but in action.

Coming Soon:

"The Untold Story of El Hadj Saad Oumar Toure"

This book is only the beginning. My next journey will take us into the **legacy of a visionary, a teacher, and a leader** whose impact has shaped generations.

El Hadj Saad Oumar Toure was more than an educator—he was a man of conviction, wisdom, and foresight. His journey was marked by challenges, resistance, and ultimately, an unwavering determination to create change.

The Untold Story of El Hadj Saad Oumar Toure is a tribute to his life, his struggles, and his enduring influence. **Stay connected** for updates as I bring his story to the world.

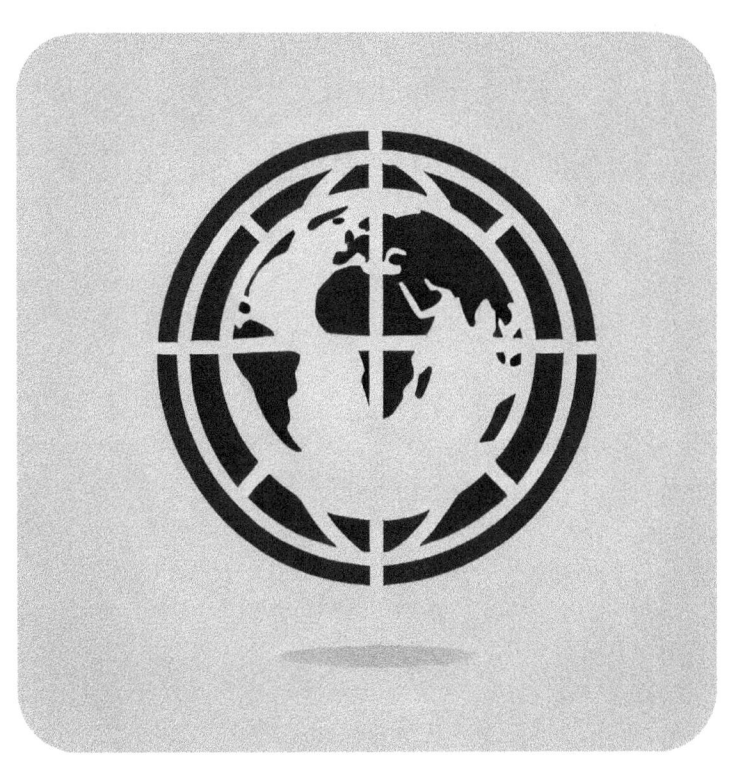

Motherhood is universal—its impact reaches far beyond any culture or country.

www.ingramcontent.com/pod-product-compliance
Lightning Source LLC
Chambersburg PA
CBHW060533030426
42337CB00021B/4244